First, the facts ...

1. Cutaneous squamous cell carcinoma (cSCC) is typically treated with surgery, without the need for other treatment.

2. cSCCs that are large, have high-risk features under the microscope or come back after surgery are more likely to need additional tests or treatments.

3. A cSCC is called 'advanced' if it grows into (invades) areas below the skin or spreads to other parts of the body.

4. Diagnosis of advanced cSCC involves looking at biopsy samples of skin and lymph nodes under the microscope and also sometimes scans or images of the area.

5. Advanced cSCC is treated with surgery, radiation treatment or drugs, or a combination of these.

6. If treatment is unsuccessful, palliative care helps to relieve the symptoms of cancer.

This book aims to help you understand your options so you can talk to your doctors, nurses and medical team about your cancer and its treatment. Use the spaces on the pages to organize your notes and questions.

My main concerns

Make a note of anything you want to discuss with your doctor here ...

EASTWICK COLLEGE
JOSEPHINE HUISKING LIBRARY
RAMSEY, NEW JERSEY

What is cutaneous squamous cell carcinoma?

Cutaneous squamous cell carcinoma (shortened to cSCC) is a type of cancer that grows in the outermost layer of the skin (cutaneous = of the skin). This outer layer of skin is called the **epidermis**. It is the body's barrier against the environment.

> Squamous cells are also found in the internal lining of places such as the throat, lungs and cervix. Although these cells can develop into squamous cell carcinomas, the cancers are different from cSCC.
>
> If you read about squamous cell carcinoma, **check the information is about the skin or cutaneous type**.

cSCC and basal cell carcinoma are **non-melanoma skin cancers**. They differ from melanoma, which comes from a different kind of cell, a melanocyte.

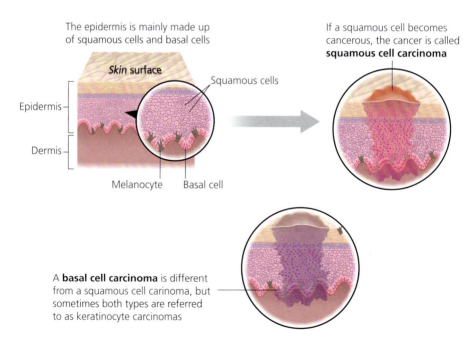

Why did I get it?

Some people are more likely to get cSCC than others – it's more common in older, fair-skinned men, for example. People who develop freckles or burn easily in the sun have a higher risk, as do people who have spent lots of time outdoors or have used indoor tanning beds.

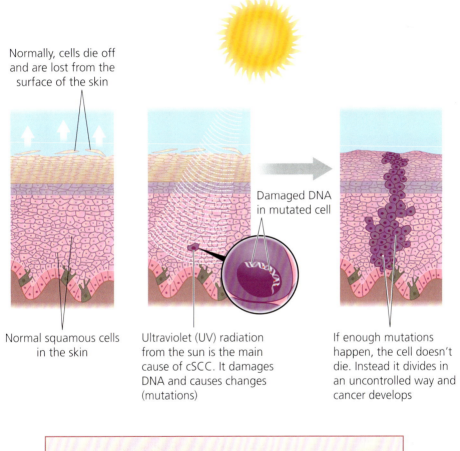

Normally, cells die off and are lost from the surface of the skin

Damaged DNA in mutated cell

Normal squamous cells in the skin

Ultraviolet (UV) radiation from the sun is the main cause of cSCC. It damages DNA and causes changes (mutations)

If enough mutations happen, the cell doesn't die. Instead it divides in an uncontrolled way and cancer develops

Some medications increase sun sensitivity and cancer risk. And some people's immune systems do not work effectively, making cSCC more likely.

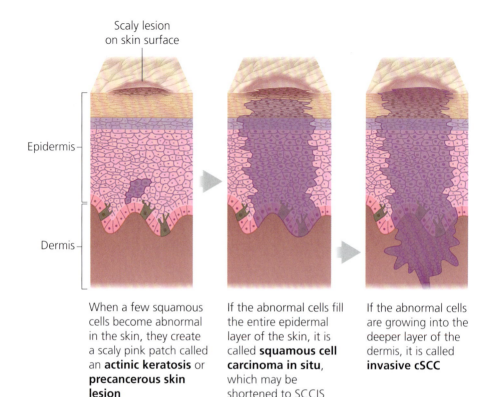

Scaly lesion on skin surface

Epidermis

Dermis

When a few squamous cells become abnormal in the skin, they create a scaly pink patch called an **actinic keratosis** or **precancerous skin lesion**

If the abnormal cells fill the entire epidermal layer of the skin, it is called **squamous cell carcinoma in situ**, which may be shortened to SCCIS

If the abnormal cells are growing into the deeper layer of the dermis, it is called **invasive cSCC**

About precancerous and cancerous lesions

Because cSCC is caused by sunlight, it is common for patients with lots of sun damage to their skin to have more than one cSCC.

Having more than one cSCC in an area of sun damage is not the same as having a cSCC that has spread to other parts of the body. We'll discuss cSCC that spreads in the next section.

Did you know?
SCC that develops inside the mouth or throat is sometimes called **head and neck SCC**, which can be easily confused with skin SCC that happens on the skin of the face, head or neck.

Questions you may have

- **Is cSCC contagious?**

    No, cSCC is not contagious – you can't catch it from someone else. And you can't spread it to anyone else, either.

- **Did I inherit cSCC from my parents?**

    The answer is less straightforward – it's yes and no.

    If you have fair skin or light-colored eyes or hair, you inherited those risk factors for cSCC from your parents. But cSCC is not usually considered to be a genetic condition.

    There are exceptions where cSCC develops because the person has a very rare genetic condition such as xeroderma pigmentosum or oculocutaneous albinism. These conditions make the person more likely to develop cSCC. But in most people, cSCC is not directly related to an inherited genetic disease.

My questions

What is advanced cSCC?

The cSCC that's diagnosed first is called a **primary cSCC**. It's usually an isolated cancer on the skin and can be removed by surgery.

But in some cases the cancer can be more aggressive and is said to be advanced. An advanced cSCC is either:

- **locally advanced**, meaning it has grown very large or is complicated to remove, or
- **metastatic**, meaning it has spread to other places.

The timeline of advanced cSCC is different for each person.

In some people, a primary cSCC is treated with surgery but the cancer later comes back in the same place; this is called a **recurrent cancer**.

Other people are diagnosed with both primary and metastatic cSCC at the same time.

And some people are diagnosed with metastatic cSCC in other parts of the body years after the primary cSCC was treated.

Local invasion

Locally advanced cSCC
Locally advanced cSCC can grow into nearby healthy areas. This may include the underlying fat, muscle or bone – it depends on the location of the cancer. The cancer can also affect a nearby body part such as an eye or an ear.

Perineural invasion
Locally advanced cSCC can also grow into the nerves of the skin or along the sleeve or sheath that surrounds nerves. This is called perineural invasion, perineural spread or perineural metastasis.

Metastatic cSCC

Why does cSCC spread?

It is rare for cSCC to spread to another place in the body. But there are some high-risk features of the primary cSCC that make this more likely, including:

- large size (over 2 cm)
- cancer recurs (comes back) in the same location after surgery
- it affects the ear or lip.

There are also some features that can be seen in the laboratory from the biopsy:

- the nerves are involved (perineural invasion – see page 6)
- the cancer cells are poorly differentiated, which means they appear spindle shaped or different from usual cancer cells
- the cancer has created a different-looking area around itself (called **desmoplasia**)
- the cancer has grown (invaded) deeply through the skin to the fat, muscle or bone underneath.

cSCC is also more likely to spread in a person whose immune system is suppressed – which happens with some conditions, such as leukemia, lymphoma and HIV/AIDS, and after an organ transplant.

What is a biopsy?

A biopsy is a procedure to remove a sample of tissue from an area. The sample can be sent to a laboratory to get more information about the types of cell in the sample – for example, a pathologist can look at them under the microscope to see what types of cell are involved.

Often, samples of lymph nodes are also taken. Lymph nodes are important collection sites for cancer cells. They can be the first place to show signs that the cancer is spreading. See page 13 for more information.

Regional and in-transit metastasis

The **lymphatic system** is made up of small vessels and lymph nodes. It runs through the body alongside blood vessels. (Lymph nodes = 'glands'.)

It's an important part of the immune system as it provides a way for immune cells to circulate around the body.

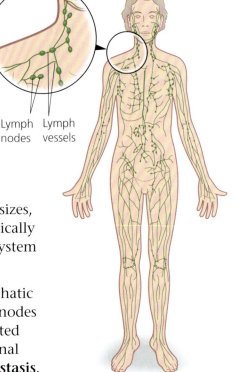

Lymph nodes   Lymph vessels

When cSCC spreads, or metastasizes, to other parts of the body, it typically travels through the lymphatic system or the bloodstream.

cSCC cells that invade the lymphatic system can travel to the lymph nodes and grow there. When the affected lymph node is close to the original tumor, it's called **regional metastasis**.

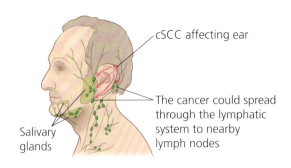

cSCC affecting ear

The cancer could spread through the lymphatic system to nearby lymph nodes

Salivary glands

Very rarely, cSCC spreads through the lymphatic system and grows in multiple tumors under the skin along the lymphatic route. This is called **in-transit metastasis**.

Distant metastasis

Distant metastasis happens when cSCC cells travel past the regional lymph nodes to lymph nodes or organs in other places in the body, as shown on the diagram:

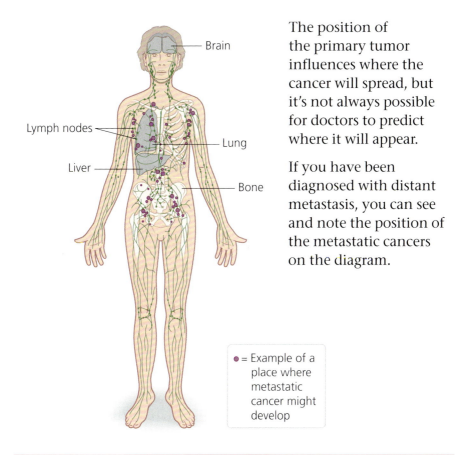

The position of the primary tumor influences where the cancer will spread, but it's not always possible for doctors to predict where it will appear.

If you have been diagnosed with distant metastasis, you can see and note the position of the metastatic cancers on the diagram.

● = Example of a place where metastatic cancer might develop

Has my cancer spread?

Diagnosis

Taking a skin biopsy for diagnosis

A primary cSCC usually appears as a new lump or sore on the skin and is diagnosed by a skin biopsy. This is a minor procedure carried out in your doctor's office, often at the same appointment as your skin check.

The doctor will clean the skin and inject a small amount of local anesthetic to numb it. A sample of the growth is removed, and the doctor will either put in a few stitches or allow the area to heal without stitches. In most cases, the biopsy is enough to make the diagnosis and plan treatment, which is normally surgery. In this case, no other tests are necessary.

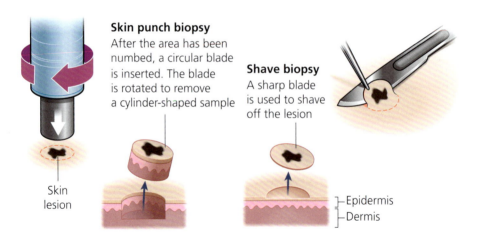

Other tests

Other tests are sometimes helpful for advanced cSCC. These are the **work up** or **staging** tests, and they can help with planning surgery. Or they may be recommended after surgery to see if more treatment is needed. Some are described on the next pages.

Imaging (scans)

The type of imaging you have depends on your individual cancer. Some people don't need it.

CT scan (= computerized tomography)
A CT scan (or sometimes 'cat scan') involves taking a series of X-rays to give a cross-sectional picture of the body. CT scans are used to see if cSCC has spread to lymph nodes or has grown into the bone.

MRI (= magnetic resonance imaging)

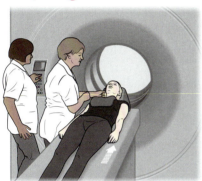

MRI builds up a picture of an area using a magnetic field. Like CT, it gives a cross-sectional picture.

PET scan (= positron emission tomography)
Before a PET scan, a radioactive tracer is delivered into a blood vessel. The tracer spreads through the body, building up at places where cancer cells are present. This is detected by the scanner. PET scans are used to see if the cancer has spread. Often a person has a PET scan and CT scan or MRI.

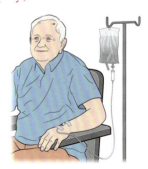

Ultrasound
Ultrasound uses high-frequency sound waves. It's used to see if cancer has spread to the lymph nodes or to check lymph nodes after surgery.

Additional biopsies

Needle biopsy

If you or your doctor feels a deeper lump under your skin, or if your imaging shows a suspicious lump in one of your lymph nodes, a needle biopsy or fine needle aspiration can be used to take a sample from the area.

The doctor will clean the skin and inject a small amount of anesthetic to numb it. If the lump is difficult to feel, he or she might use ultrasound to help find it.

A needle is put into the skin to collect a sample of cells from the lump. This may be repeated several times. Once the biopsy is complete, it will be sent to the laboratory. Ask your doctor when you can expect to hear the results.

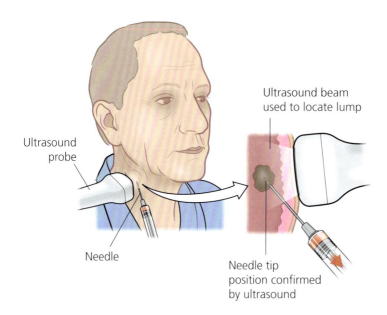

Sentinel lymph node biopsy

Sentinel lymph node biopsy is used to see whether your cSCC has spread into your lymphatic system – the **sentinel nodes** are the first lymph nodes that would be affected if your cancer is spreading.

To identify the sentinel lymph nodes, a radioactive tracer, a blue dye or both will be injected into the area of the primary cSCC. The radioactive tracer is injected a few hours or a day before surgery. The blue dye is usually injected during surgery.

The dye or tracer travels through the lymphatic system to the nearby lymph nodes. Your surgeon will detect the tracer from its radioactivity, while the dye will turn the lymph nodes blue. Once the sentinel lymph nodes have been identified, one or more will be removed and sent to the laboratory to look for tumor cells.

The risks of this procedure depend on the position of your cancer and the lymph nodes.

Talk to your surgeon about what it might mean for you.

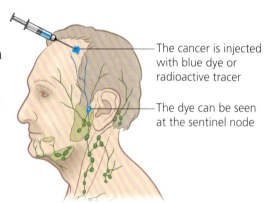

The cancer is injected with blue dye or radioactive tracer

The dye can be seen at the sentinel node

Removing other lymph nodes in the area

If you are having a sentinel lymph node biopsy or have signs of cSCC in your lymph nodes, your surgeons will discuss whether the other lymph nodes in the area should be removed completely.

Staging

Cancer staging is a way of describing how much a cancer has grown or spread. Staging your cSCC will help your medical team share information with you about treatment options and your outlook.

cSCC is staged using a system called TNM:

- **T** describes how advanced your **T**umor is, from T1 (least advanced) to T4 (most advanced).
- **N** describes whether your cSCC has spread to your lymph **N**odes: N1 or higher means your lymph nodes contain cancer.
- **M** describes any **M**etastatic cancer at places other than the lymph nodes: M1 means the cSCC has spread.

Your T, N and M scores are combined into your overall stage. Tumor in situ or Tis means there are abnormal cells present, but the cancerous cells are confined to the epidermal layer and have not invaded the dermis.

Working out the cancer stage

T score: if the tumor…	T score is:
fills the epidermal layer of the skin	Tis
is 2 cm or less in size	T1
is more than 2 cm but no larger than 4 cm	T2
is over 4 cm or is starting to affect bone or nearby nerves, has grown through the fat layer under the skin or is deeper than 6 mm	T3
is growing into the bone	T4

> **Staging procedures are not always needed**
> Not all cSCCs need imaging or sentinel lymph node biopsy – it depends on the initial features. If the risk of the cancer spreading is low, it may be that the risks of imaging or biopsy outweigh any benefit.

N score: are the lymph nodes affected?	N score is:
No	N0
One node affected, same side, not larger than 3 cm and no spread outside the node	N1
One node affected, same side, not larger than 3 cm but has started to spread outside the node, *OR* One node, same side, between 3 cm and 6 cm but no spread outside the node	N2a
More than one node affected, same side, none larger than 6 cm and no spread outside the nodes	N2b
More than one node affected, both sides or opposite side, none larger than 6 cm and no spread outside the nodes	N2c
Larger than 6 cm but no spread outside the node(s)	N3a
One node affected, same side, larger than 3 cm and has started to spread outside the node, *OR* Several nodes (same side, opposite side or both sides) affected and at least one has spread outside the node, *OR* A node affected on opposite side and has started to spread outside the node	N3b

Guide to the wording

Same side (ipsilateral): node on same side of the body as the cancer

Opposite side (contralateral): node on opposite side of the body to the cancer

Both sides (bilateral): nodes on both sides of the body

Spread outside the node: starting to grow into the fatty layer around the node

M score: has the cancer spread to a different place in the body?	M score is:
No	M0
Yes	M1

When T is:	And N is:	And M is:	The cancer is stage:
Tis	N0	M0	0
T1	N0	M0	I
T2	N0	M0	II
T3	N0	M0	III
T1	N1	M0	III
T2	N1	M0	III
T3	N1	M0	III
T1	N2	M0	IV
T2	N2	M0	IV
T3	N2	M0	IV
Any T	N3	M0	IV
T4	Any N	M0	IV
Any T	Any N	M1	IV

My cancer TNM scores and stage

T: N: M: Stage:

Features of my cancer

Make a note here about any individual features of your cancer that your doctor has told you about (for example, position or spread) ...

My cancer timeline

Make a note here about your cancer development if it will be helpful (for example, is it a recurrence?) ...

My questions

If you think of any questions you'd like to ask your doctor, note them here ...

Surgery

Wide local excision

The aim of wide local excision is to remove the cancer and an area of normal skin around the cancer, and then reconstruct the skin and surrounding area.

The area of normal skin is called the **margin** and it is sent to the laboratory to check for signs of cancer. If the margin is clear, it is likely that all the cancer has been removed. The pathologist will also check for high-risk features in samples of the cancer (see page 7).

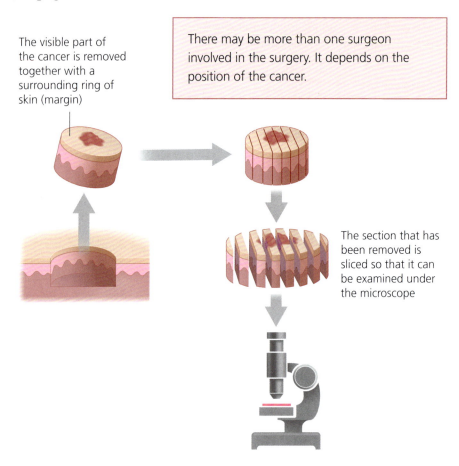

The visible part of the cancer is removed together with a surrounding ring of skin (margin)

There may be more than one surgeon involved in the surgery. It depends on the position of the cancer.

The section that has been removed is sliced so that it can be examined under the microscope

Mohs micrographic surgery

Mohs micrographic surgery is used for some locally advanced cancers. During surgery, layers of skin are removed and checked for cancer. This continues until all the cancer has been removed.

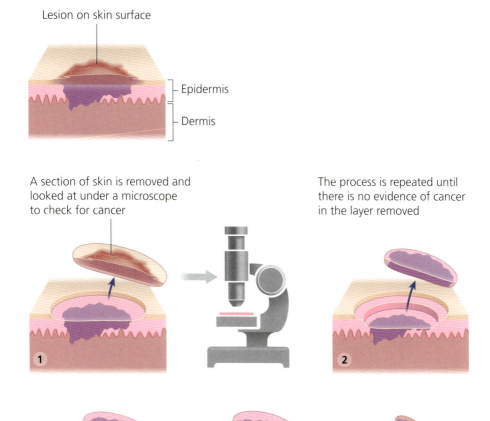

Radiation therapy (radiotherapy)

Sessions of radiation therapy might be recommended:

- to prevent advanced cSCC from returning after it has been completely removed with surgery (**adjuvant therapy**), or
- to treat any remaining cancer cells if the cancer cannot be completely removed with surgery, or
- to treat advanced cSCC that cannot be treated with surgery (**definitive therapy**), or
- if it can help relieve pain or symptoms of incurable cSCC (**palliative radiation**).

First, a customized mask or mold is made. This is worn during each treatment so that you are in the same position every time. Then images are taken and treatment is planned. Tiny markings or tattoos may be needed to make sure you are in the same position every time.

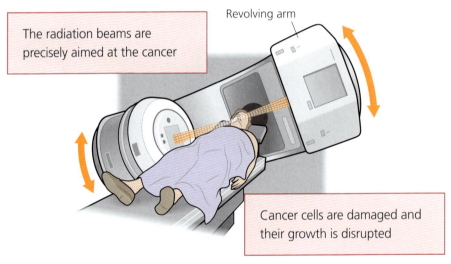

The radiation beams are precisely aimed at the cancer

Revolving arm

Cancer cells are damaged and their growth is disrupted

Side effects

Side effects can include fatigue, loss of appetite, skin changes or hair loss. If your head or neck is involved, you may develop mouth sores, changes in taste, tooth decay or trouble swallowing.

Systemic treatment

Systemic treatment is needed if cSCC has spread throughout the body (see pages 7–9). Your treatment will be prescribed by a specialist in medical cancer treatment (oncologist). Talk to your oncologist about your treatment options, and the risks and benefits of each choice.

Chemotherapy kills cancer cells directly

Potential side effects include: nausea, vomiting, loss of appetite, hair loss, fatigue, anemia (low level of red blood cells), risk of infection, hearing changes/ringing in ears, neuropathy (numbness and tingling in hands and feet)

Targeted molecular inhibitors kill cells by blocking specific cancer behaviors

Potential side effects include: rash, eye changes, diarrhea, nausea, decreased appetite, constipation, neutropenia (low white blood cell counts), risk of infection, liver problems, lung problems

Immunotherapy overcomes the way cancer hides from the body's immune system so the body's immune defenses work against the cancer cells

Potential side effects include: fatigue, rash, diarrhea, nausea, decreased appetite, constipation, muscle aches, autoimmune problems

Tell your doctor about any changes – side effects vary from person to person

Questions to ask your doctor about your treatment

If you're having **surgery**:

- What are the risks of this procedure?
- Should I stop any of my medications before surgery?
- What can I expect after my surgery?
- Will I need help at home during my recovery?

If you're having **radiation therapy**:

- What are the risks of radiation?
- How many treatments will I have?
- What can I expect during my radiation therapy?
- Will I need help at home?

If you're having **systemic treatment**:

- Which treatment is right for me?
- Will I have to come to the hospital for intravenous treatment? How often?
- How will we know if the treatment is working?
- How will I feel during treatment?
- Will I need help at home?

My questions

Make a note of any questions you have for your doctor here ...

What can I do to help myself?

Taking care of the mind and body can help during cancer treatment and recovery.

Whatever you do, do it in moderation. Always ask your doctor if you are concerned.

- Eat a balanced and varied diet of healthy vegetables, fruits, chicken and fish – cut down on fats, carbs and sweets.

- Try to exercise regularly – even a daily walk will help your physical strength (if you have challenges with walking and balance, discuss this with your doctor).

- Continue to check your skin for new lesions, and protect yourself from the sun with sunscreen, hats and clothing.

- Get outdoors – fresh air and sunlight (with sunscreen, of course!) will have a positive effect on your mood.

- If you smoke, try to cut down or stop.

- If your doctor says that it's ok to drink alcohol, do so in moderation.

- Consider meditation, yoga or relaxation techniques to calm the mind if you are feeling stressed.

- Find small things to be appreciative of every day.

- If you are religious, your community can help support you.

- Think about joining a support group – it's helpful to talk to other people going through the same thing; find details on the internet or ask your cancer center.

Palliative care

If your disease becomes untreatable, you will be referred to a palliative care team. A comprehensive assessment can highlight issues or problems beyond any specific symptoms, such as social difficulties or concerns about future care. A wide range of support is available.

End of life care

A lot can be done to help your symptoms in the final stages of cancer. But it is important to have open and honest discussions with your medical team, family and friends, and anyone else involved in your care so that your expectations are realistic. You will need to make your preferences for future care known. This includes the care you would like to receive toward the end of life and life-sustaining treatments.

Your feelings

There is no right or wrong way to feel about your illness and the future, but it may help to:

- focus on what is important to you
- spend time with your loved ones
- make plans ahead of time for you and your family
- keep to your usual routines to maintain a sense of normality
- accept that there will be good days and bad days
- ask your medical team about options for social and emotional support as well as physical support.

Research

For skin cancers, research is looking at:

- new treatments, such as targeted molecular inhibitors and immunotherapies (see page 21)
- improving methods of imaging to improve skin biopsy
- developing new ways of diagnosing cSCC and predicting how it will develop.

Research into cSCC could not happen without people:

- taking part in clinical trials of new treatments
- donating blood or tissue samples for research
- raising funds for research organizations at their own hospital or nationally.

If you would like to be more involved in research, discuss the possibilities with your medical team or contact a skin cancer organization or charity.

Clinical trials

New therapies for cancer are evolving all the time. One of the ways people can access new treatments is by taking part in a clinical trial. Ask your oncologist if there is a clinical trial that is right for you and discuss the risks and benefits of taking part.

If you want to learn more about clinical trials for your cSCC, visit www.clinicaltrials.gov, www.clinicaltrialsregister.eu, www.anzctr.org.au or search 'clinical trials database'.

My notes on research

Write notes or questions about research trials here ...

Asking questions

Everyone deals with cancer differently. You may want to collect detailed information and research your cancer, or you may prefer to trust your medical team to guide you. Being informed will help you have better conversations and make decisions about your treatment and care.

Some conversations with your doctor may involve a lot of new information and questions. Bringing a family member or friend and taking notes can help you to take in this information and make decisions.

Ask the questions that are bothering you, and if you are not sure about any aspect of your treatment, ask again. Don't be afraid to ask for a second opinion – it's absolutely acceptable.

Make a note below of the health professionals in your medical team.

Name	Specialty or role	Contact information

Useful resources

American Academy of Dermatology
www.aad.org

American Cancer Society
www.cancer.org/cancer/basal-and-squamous-cell-skin-cancer.html

American College of Mohs Surgery
www.skincancermohssurgery.org

American Skin Association
www.americanskin.org

British Association of Dermatologists' patient information
www.skinhealthinfo.org.uk/condition/squamous-cell-carcinomas

British Skin Foundation
www.britishskinfoundation.org.uk

Cancer Research UK
www.cancerresearchuk.org

International Cancer Information Service Group members
https://icisg.org/membership/membership-list

National Cancer Institute (USA)
www.cancer.gov/types/skin

Skin Cancer Foundation (USA)
www.skincancer.org

U.S. National Institutes of Health clinical trials database
www.clinicaltrials.gov

Glossary

Actinic keratosis: scaly pink patch of skin formed by abnormal squamous cells (sometimes called a precancerous skin lesion)

Basal cell carcinoma: a cancer that develops from a basal cell (rather than a squamous cell, as happens in cSCC)

Biopsy: a procedure to remove a sample of tissue so that its features can be investigated

Clinical trial: a study involving people designed to answer a specific question about a treatment

cSCC: the shortened way of saying cutaneous squamous cell carcinoma

CT scan: CT is the shortened way of saying computerized tomography. A CT scan is a three-dimensional picture or image of the area that a computer creates from multiple X-ray images

Dermis: a deeper layer of the skin that lies below the epidermis

Epidermis: the outer layer of skin

Invasive: a cancer is invasive if it has spread out of the area in which it developed and is growing into surrounding healthy areas

Locally advanced: a cancer is locally advanced if it is growing into nearby healthy areas

Lymph node: a nodule that's part of the body's lymphatic system. The nodes filter the fluid that travels through the lymphatic system (called lymph). They also contain white blood cells that fight infections. There are hundreds of lymph nodes in the lymphatic system

Margin: the apparently normal edge or border of skin (or other tissue) that is removed in surgery for cancer. It is checked for cancer cells – if there are no cancer cells present, the margin is said to be clear or negative, and if there are cancer cells, it is said to be involved or positive

Melanoma: a cancer that develops from a melanocyte or other cell type that produces pigment (rather than a squamous cell, as happens in cSCC)

Metastasis: when cancer cells break away from the original tumor, travel to another place in the body via the blood or lymphatic system and a new tumor develops

Mohs micrographic surgery: a surgical procedure in which the area is removed in layers that are then checked for signs of cancer; the layers continue to be removed while there are still signs of cancer present

MRI: the shortened way of saying magnetic resonance imaging. A computer produces detailed pictures of areas inside the body from signals generated by radio waves and a magnet

Perineural invasion: when cancer spreads into the nerves

PET scan: PET is the shortened way of saying positron emission tomography. A small amount of radioactive tracer is injected into a vein and then builds up at the cancer sites. These areas then show up on the scan images

Radiation therapy: the use of high-energy radiation from X-rays, gamma rays, neutrons, protons and other sources to stop cancer cells from growing and dividing

Recurrence: when a cancer returns after being undetectable for a time following treatment

SCC in situ: when the abnormal squamous cells fill the epidermis layer

Sentinel lymph node: the most likely lymph node to be first affected by cancer that is spreading

Stage: the extent of cancer in the body

Systemic therapy: treatment with cancer drugs that travel in the blood and reach all the cancer cells around the body

Sources used in the preparation of this document

American Joint Committee on Cancer. *AJCC Cancer Staging Form Supplement. AJCC Cancer Staging Manual*, 8th edn. Chicago: AJCC, 2018.

Bolognia JL, Schaffer JV, Cerroni L, eds. *Dermatology*, 4th edn. Philadelphia: London, 2017.

Chen L, Aria AB, Silapunt S, Migden MR. Emerging nonsurgical therapies for locally advanced and metastatic nonmelanoma skin cancer. *Dermatol Surg* 2019;45:1–16.

Koyfman SA, Cooper JS, Beitler JJ et al. ACR Appropriateness Criteria(®) aggressive nonmelanomatous skin cancer of the head and neck. *Head Neck* 2016;38:175–82.

Que SKT, Zwald FO, Schmults CD. Cutaneous squamous cell carcinoma: incidence, risk factors, diagnosis, and staging. *J Am Acad Dermatol* 2018;78: 237–47.

Schmults CD, Blitzblau R, Aasi SZ et al. NCCN clinical practice guidelines in oncology (NCCN Guidelines®) squamous cell skin cancer; version 1.2020 2 October 2019, National Comprehensive Cancer Network Inc. Available at NCCN.org (registration required). A patient version is available at www.nccn.org/patients/guidelines/squamous_cell/index.html.

Tolkachjov SN, Brodland DG, Coldiron BM et al. Understanding Mohs micrographic surgery: a review and practical guide for the nondermatologist. *Mayo Clin Proc* 2017;92:1261–71.

Trodello C, Pepper JP, Wong M, Wysong A. Cisplatin and cetuximab treatment for metastatic cutaneous squamous cell carcinoma: a systematic review. *Dermatol Surg* 2017;43:40–9.

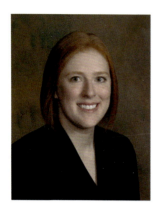

Authored by **Dr Sarah Arron** MD PhD

Assistant Professor of Dermatology
Director, High Risk Skin Cancer Program
Chief of Mohs Micrographic Surgery, San Francisco
Veterans Administration Medical Center
University of California, San Francisco
CA, USA

© 2020 in this edition S. Karger Publishers Limited
ISBN: 978-1-912776-36-8

Questions for the Editor

What have you found the most useful about this book? What is missing? Do you still have any unanswered questions? Please send your questions, or any other comments, to fastfacts@karger.com and help future readers of future editions. Thank you!

With sincere thanks to those who have reviewed this publication for all their help and guidance